THE FOETAL CIRCULATION

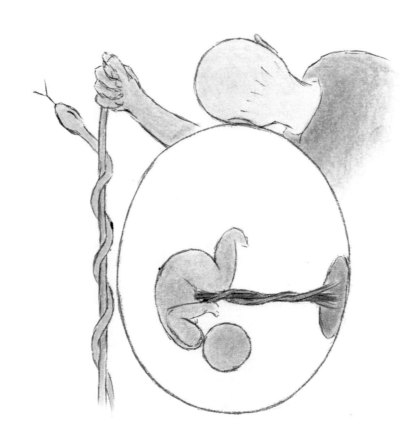

7th edition

Alan Gilchrist

AuthorHouse™ UK
1663 Liberty Drive
Bloomington, IN 47403 USA
www.authorhouse.co.uk
UK TFN: 0800 0148641 (Toll Free inside the UK)
UK Local: 02036 956322 (+44 20 3695 6322 from outside the UK)

This book is printed on acid-free paper.

ISBN: 978-1-6655-9130-0 (sc)
ISBN: 978-1-6655-9129-4 (e)

Print information available on the last page.

Published by AuthorHouse 08/20/2021

authorHOUSE®

Contents

Dedication.

This seventh edition is specially dedicated to the memory of Pauline, and to the four children she gave us, Peter Andrew Elizabeth and Mary.

Acknowledgements.

First and foremost, I am very grateful to my son Andrew who keeps an eye on me and keeps me alive by doing my weekly shopping. I must thank Sophia Anderton again for allowing me to publish data from the British Journal of Radiology in the 6th edition, a small part of which is included in this one. John Quinn has again come out of retirement to help with the reproduction and placing of the diagrams and pictures, and I thank him sincerely for his dedicated work.

Between 1953 and 1963, prosperous Northern and Southern Rhodesia were joined with Nyasaland to form the Central African Federation of Rhodesia and Nyasaland, to help Nyasaland with few natural resources. The story I am about to relate begins in Bulawayo, Southern Rhodesia, now called Zimbabwe, when I went there in December 1954. After seven and a half years in Nyasaland, now known as Malawi, I returned to Southern Rhodesia in 1963, and the story ends there in 1969. The events in Nyasaland may seem to have no bearing on the foetal circulation, but I consider them to be steppingstones back to Rhodesia where I uncovered its long- hidden secrets.

I first became interested in the foetal circulation in a biology lesson when I was a medical student and heard about two different streams of blood in the right atrium of the foetal heart. I pricked up my ears, I did not doubt it but wondered how it was done. Some years later after qualification, during my National Service, I was returning to England from Malaya in a troopship in the middle of the Indian Ocean and decided on a career in plastic surgery. First, I would do a year in pathology, and then house jobs in medicine and surgery before attempting to climb the surgical ladder. After the pathology year in Nottingham General Hospital, I became a house physician in the Darlington Memorial Hospital, before doing six months in Canterbury as a house surgeon. The pathologist in Canterbury knew I had done the pathology job; he had a pathologist friend in Bulawayo with his own laboratory who wanted an assistant. Would I be interested? I eventually accepted, it led to 15 extraordinary years in Africa as a government medical officer, and an affection for the African people. It also led to my finding the answer to the riddle of the two streams, which I will tell you about if you will be patient and read the first part of my story first.

Main Street Bulawayo 1957. (Taken when I was on sick leave).

Note the wide streets. Cecil Rhodes said they had to be wide enough to let an ox wagon turn round.

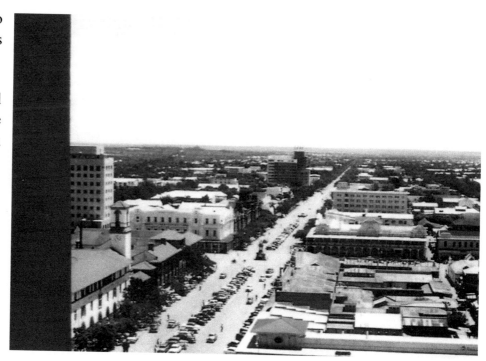

The 'path' job did not work out; I think he expected an older and more experienced man, and I expected a less disgruntled and more friendly one. The work was well within my compass, the hours were good, and the pay was more than a houseman's. I was able to buy a car and enjoy playing tennis on the sand courts in and around Bulawayo. I knew I would have to leave at the end of my year's contract and began to study for surgery again. There was a book on embryology in the lab and it contained the same idea of two different streams in the same chamber of the heart. When I got the sack in December 1955, I did not want to crawl home with my tail between my legs, I wanted to see Lake Nyasa and work with the African people up north. I drove up to Salisbury the capital, now called Harare, and met Richard Morris the first Federal Secretary for Health. I said if he would send me up to Nyasaland, I would join the government medical service. He offered me Fort Johnston, at the south end of the lake, and I gladly accepted. I spent three weeks holiday travelling round South Africa to Cape Town, Durban and Johannesburg, before beginning my new job in Salisbury on 1st January 1956, and after several weeks' training I was on my way up north in my little Morris station wagon.

Fort Johnston.

Fort Johnston was a small township on the west side of the river Shire, pronounced like cheery, five miles south of the bar, where the river flowed southwards and joined the Zambezi. The 'calendar lake' as it was called, was magnificent and beautiful, 365 miles long and 52 miles wide at the widest point. The water was fresh and potable with an abundance of beautiful edible fish. We were in the rift valley, and although the altitude was 1500 feet above sea level, we were low compared with the central African region, and it was hot throughout most of the year. In the Fort there were government offices with a district commissioner in the Colonial Service, and three assistant district commissioners, all of whom were university graduates. The small hospital had male and female wards and a maternity wing, and there was an operating theatre which had electricity from the town's generator.

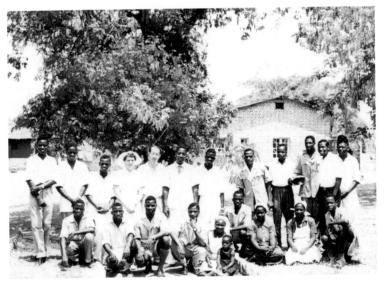

The staff consisted of a British sister, an African principal medical assistant, several African medical aides and an African midwife, plus the doctor, all seen in this picture.

There was a small club, with a concrete tennis court, a snooker table with a rather worn cloth and a different sort of bar.

The picture shows the police officer and his wife playing tennis in the cool of an early Sunday morning.

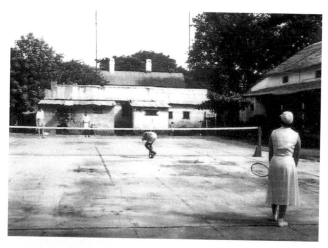

100 yards from the hospital compound was my house, seen here with me and my car, a big double storey affair, gauzed in against mosquitoes. The 'garden' at the back ran down to the Shire where crocs and hippos abounded. I never saw any of them but heard the hippos each night when they foraged and splashed around making their terrible grunts and bellows at the bottom of the garden. I gave hospitality one night to a small family passing through the Fort and told them not to be worried about the hippo noises. I could imitate the double noise they made quite well and gave them an imitation. The parents slept in the room next to mine, and in between was a small connecting room where the little girl slept. In the night the hippos obliged beautifully, and I heard the little girl say "Mummy, was that Dr Gilchrist?"

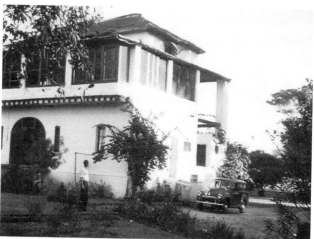

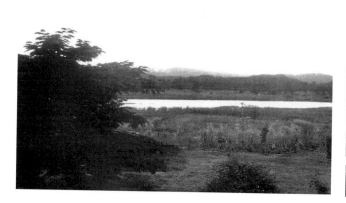

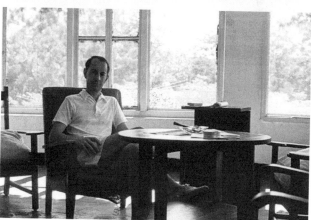

The picture on the left shows the river Shire at the bottom of my 'garden.' On the right is the upstairs verandah which was my living room. Note the shorts and the naughty pipe and tobacco tin.

We did not eat well at the Fort, at least I as a bachelor did not. My servant made the bread, and the paraffin friges struggled to keep cool the milk made from powder. I lost weight and on two occasions was admitted to Zomba hospital eighty miles away, first in 1957 with hepatitis and later with severe diarrhoea and vomiting.

The Fort Johnston District was large, probably the largest in the country with an area of about 3000 square miles, or half the size of Yorkshire. There were seven dispensaries, scattered in all directions, each with a medical aide in charge and stocked up with medicines, three of them being 60 miles away from the Fort. Eventually, I visited them all in turn each Friday by Land Rover. The medical aides knew when it was their turn and kept the patients aside they wanted me to see. Those needing hospital treatment came back with me, and sometimes we returned with the Land Rover packed full in the dark.

Our work was of the widest spectrum; there were caesarean sections, ruptured uteruses, intestinal obstructions, fractures, inguinal hernias, croc and hippo bites, puff adder bites and the tropical diseases malaria, schistosomiasis and hookworm which caused severe anaemia. We had no blood, no x-rays, no mobile phones and no HIV. The principal medical assistant, Mr Kulemaka, was a good man who was competent to cope with many of the diseases. I learned a lot from him. The general anaesthetic for my operations, after an injection of atropine as a pre-med, was an induction by ethyl chloride sprayed on to a Schimmelbusch mask, followed by ether dropped on to the mask, usually administered by the medical assistant. With some of the inguinal hernias I only used local anaesthetic. We had a few births with congenital abnormalities, two of them seen here, with hare lip, and amelia with the baby born without arms. We also delivered a rare case of ectopia vesicae, not shown here, with the bladder opening outside onto the front of the abdomen.

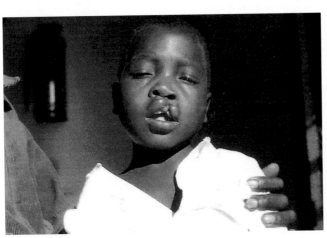

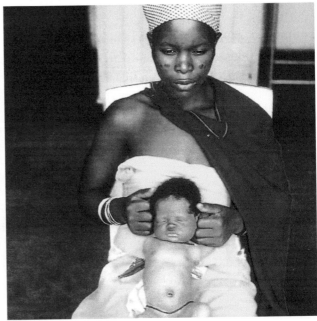

It was not long before Mr Kulemaka was replaced by Silas D Kumsinda, another good man. I began to learn Cinyanja, the language of Nyasaland, and Mr Kumsinda came into my house weekly and taught me most ably, with all the grammar and the tenses etc.

We checked the haemoglobin levels on our hospital patients weekly, and on one occasion all the patients were anaemic. I put the adults on iron pills daily and the children on syrup. I asked the officer in charge of medical stores in Zomba for Imferon. He had never heard of it but imported some for me. I then gave the adults with less than 50% haemoglobin one injection each week, and those with less than 20% an injection twice a week. The results were interesting, which ever route was used, injection pills or syrup, all the patients improved by 10% each week. Imferon became popular but iron injections were unnecessary, except perhaps for those patients we lost track of who would have had a depot of iron to continue the treatment.

At the end of 1957, I took home leave and lived with my parents, staying for three weeks in the guest wing of East Grinstead hospital and watched the surgeons performing their plastic surgery. I did not see a cleft lip repaired but attended a lecture on the subject and made careful notes. I was able buy all the instruments required and took them back to the Fort.

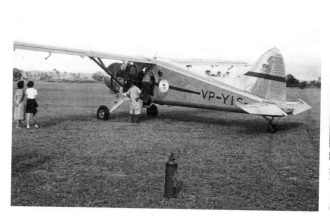 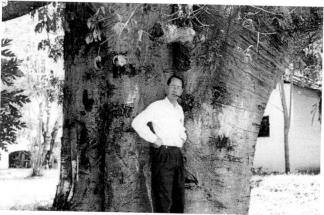

We had an airstrip at the Fort with a weekly service from Blantyre by a Canadian de havilland Beaver. Note our firefighting equipment.

On my last day in Fort Johnston, I scratched my initials and 1956-59 on a baobab tree in the garden and a visiting priest took this picture.

Blantyre.

In early 1959 I was posted to Blantyre and worked in the new Federal Queen Elizabeth Hospital. I learned a lot there, including how to perform endo-tracheal intubation and use short and long- acting muscle relaxants. I also learned how to do the lower segment caesarean section, which became of great benefit for my future African ladies in difficult labour. To my shame I must confess that I had only used the classical method at the Fort. After six months in Blantyre, I was posted to Dedza in the Central Province.

Dedza

Dedza was the antithesis of Fort Johnston. It was in a small district high up in the cool Angoni Highlands of the Central Province on the western side of the lake. In the short winter we had fires in our homes. The houses were not supplied with electricity, and we used paraffin pressure lamps for illumination. The postmaster had secretly connected the post-office generator to our hospital theatre, and we always had lights there. The Angoni and Achewa staff were friendly and respectful, and we got on very well. They spoke Cinyanja nicely, and I was able to resume my study of the language. On 24th March 1960 I passed the oral and written parts of the advanced examination.

This picture of the Dedza staff brings back the fondest memories of my work in Africa. In no other job, before or since, was I as happy as I had been in Dedza. A happy family.

We began to see ruptured ectopic pregnancies in Deza, about one a month. I had seen none in the Fort.

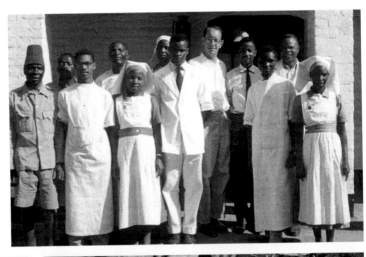

I had not been long in Dedza when there was an outbreak of smallpox in one of the villages.

On my first visit I saw 56 cases. On the next visit I brought my camera and took some photos. Two of them show the girls with the rash, while the third shows a later healed stage known locally as Ntomba.

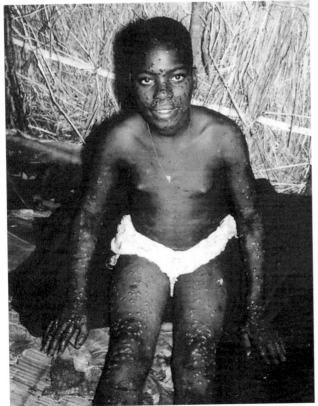

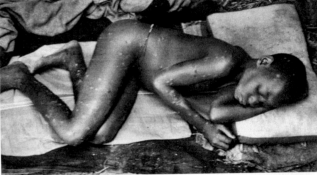

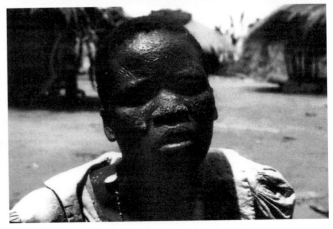

One day the hospital cook brought his son to me with a large hare lip on the right side. I revised the East Grinstead lecture, took him to theatre and intubated him through the nose, while the anaesthetic was thiopentone. I took several pictures afterwards including the three shown here, but had not taken one before, so I have reversed the earlier left sided one to show you what the pre-op condition would have looked like.

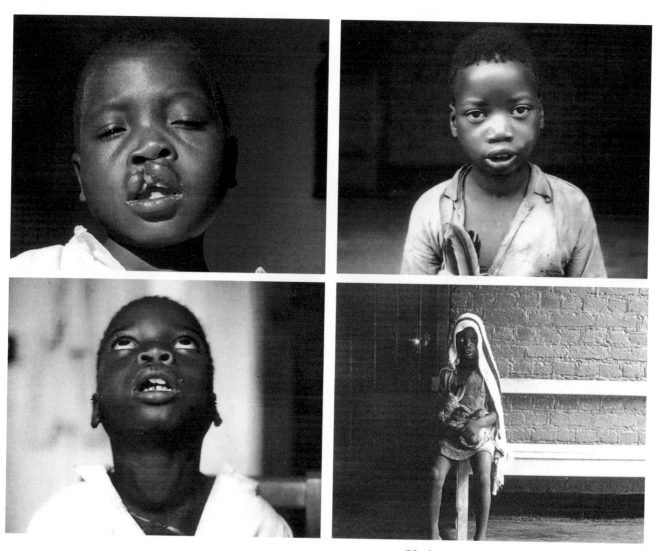

He brought me a chicken.

Shortly afterwards a young man appeared with an ugly double cleft lip. I took pictures and took him to theatre, broke the upper gums, the maxillae, with a blunt instrument, pushed them back into place and repaired the lip as best I could. The result was not perfect but an improvement.

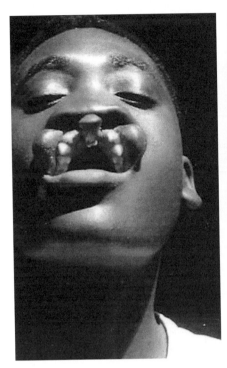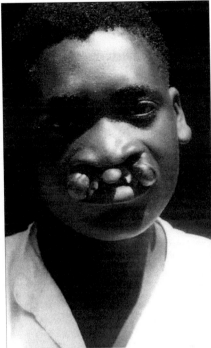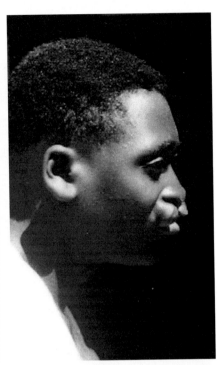

When he came back later, he told me he had got married.

The Federal government had given each of the three territories an A level boarding school for African students. In Nyasaland the school was in the healthy district of Dedza, on the other side of Dedza mountain. I did not visit the school, but I treated some of the students. We admitted one of them who was very ill, and the laboratory assistant showed me a tube of his blood which was almost completely haemolised, leaving the red cells at the bottom of the tube below the clear serum. I was powerless to help him, and he died of blackwater fever, the only case I had seen, in an African student in high up healthy Dedza.

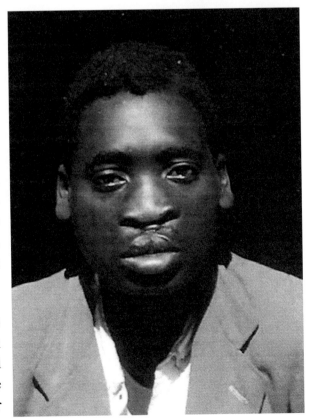

One night the medical assistant sent the messenger to me with a note telling me there was a ruptured uterus in the hospital and he could hear the foetal heart. I dashed to the hospital and delivered a live baby; part of the placenta was still attached to the torn uterus. Another rare case. Top marks for the medical assistant, Green Nyrenda, a Tumbuka from the Northern Province.

Mzuzu.

At the end of 1960 I was posted to the Northern Province as Provincial Medical Officer and stationed at Mzuzu. Three times I visited Karonga at the far north, once by car and twice by the Beaver. Throughout my stay in Nyasaland there had been increasing unrest, aggravated by the arrival of Dr Banda. A state of emergency had been declared in 1959 and Banda and many others had been detained or imprisoned. The Federation was to be dismantled and elections were held to decide who should lead the Future independent Malawi. I saw the voting taking place in Mzuzu in election tents.

After three pleasant months in Mzuzu I was posted to Lilongwe as Medical Officer in Charge.

Lilongwe

The European and African hospitals in Lilongwe were the third busiest in the Federation after Salisbury and Bulawayo, and we had only three doctors. I did the surgery and the admin, another with the higher qualification of MRCP looked after the medical cases, and the third worked in the maternity unit. We had an x-ray machine and a lady to work it. Things were always happening in Lilongwe, the first occurred soon after I had arrived there. Returning late from a court case in Blantyre I was assaulted by a thug who knocked me out unconscious. He damaged my nose and I had to have surgery on it later when I was on home leave. The next was the arrival of a young African doctor who had been posted to join us. He was a fine young gentleman who had qualified from Fort Hare University in South Africa, and he was accompanied by his lovely wife and their two children, a boy and a girl. He entertained me in his house with singing and guitar playing. He joined me in theatre and showed me how to treat a fractured shaft of femur with an intra-medullary nail. He had seen it done in Salisbury. I gave him half my outpatient clinics. There was no problem with the African or Asian, but the local white farmers objected when it came to the European. The first I knew about it was when I was confronted in my office by two of the farmers and a group of officials from medical headquarters in Salisbury. I had to rescind the arrangement, and our fourth doctor was posted to Port Herald on the lower Shire. He later became a successful pathologist with his own laboratory in Harare. The smallpox followed us up to Lilongwe and I vaccinated his son. I suppose the scar is still visible. The ectopics followed us up to Lilongwe like the smallpox, and I had to operate on a white lady whom I had known in the Fort. I also did my only white caesarean in Lilongwe, noted not for the colour of her skin, but because it was the first and only time that I had opened the bladder. I stitched it up and we put in a catheter and the patient was charming about it. But one of the sisters objected strongly when I described my mistake in the notes which were clearly visible in the duty room frequented by staff and patients alike. I relented, turned the notes round so that my error was not to be seen and kept everyone happy. We were paid a visit by a team of three from Makerere in Uganda led by an English surgeon Denis Burkitt who were investigating the distribution of a strange tumour which affected the facial skeleton of African children. I had seen cases on a ferry crossing the Shire down river. There was a training school in Lilongwe for female medical aides, and the doctors helped with the lectures. In my first lecture the sister in charge, who was the wife of the doctor with the Membership, came in with the trainees and sat behind them. I began by telling them about my experience with the treatment of anaemia in Fort Johnston. When I told them that the injections were unnecessary the sister blurted out "Blathers." I explained that they had been my own observations. "Blathers." She said again rudely. The lecture broke up in disarray. Later, she and her husband were posted to Northern Rhodesia where he probably became the medical specialist there.

My last story from Lilongwe concerns the young son of an African police officer who had jumped into a rubbish pit, not knowing that the ashes underneath were glowing hot. Both legs were badly burned, and in spite of all our efforts to save him he continued to lose condition and go downhill. Grafting may have aggravated the loss of fluid. During my stay in East Grinstead I learned that grafts taken from a close relative could survive for up to six or eight weeks. So, we took him and his mother to theatre, anaesthetised both on either side of me and I took large grafts from her legs. I cut them up into several pieces postage stamp size and applied them to his raw areas. The grafts survived until his own regenerated skin took over and he turned the corner and made a good recovery.

Zomba

After a year in Lilongwe, I was posted to Zomba, the capital, as Medical Superintendent in charge of the African and European hospitals. There were four of us doctors and sometimes we had a fifth. Although my work was administrative, I did my fair share of the medical work and took it in turns to be on call for emergencies. I also ran a daily outpatients' clinic for the Europeans. The Federation was coming to an end, and I met some interesting people there. Some were destined to be governors of the remnants of the Empire which still existed in other far- flung places in the world. I began to meet some of the new African

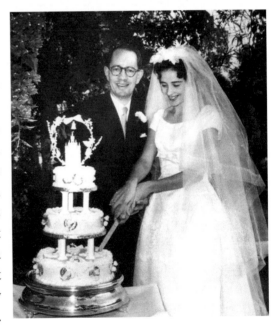

leaders of the country who had been given houses formerly occupied by Europeans. There was an active amateur drama group in Zomba with some talented members. The Minister for Finance put on 'The Yeomen of the Guard', and I joined in as one of the bearded yeomen. Near me was a young pretty maid in the chorus whose beautiful eyes always seemed to be coming in my direction, and mine in hers I suppose. She shared her sandwiches with me in the interval of the dress rehearsal, and after the public performance I fell madly in love with her. She was Pauline, the daughter of a local farmer and businessman, and had been born in Zomba hospital 21 years previously. The following year we were married on 17th August 1963 and left immediately after the reception for Rhodesia where I had been offered the post of medical superintendent of Fort Victoria hospital. We travelled in two cars with my servant and his wife and young son, plus a dog and three cats.

My several appointments in Nyasaland deserve a summary. They all took place in a part of Africa I had chosen and loved. Most of my patients had been Africans who had put their trust in a stranger from England, though often they had had no option. I enjoyed working with them. They were born strong and led lives which developed their strength, but some were afflicted with diseases and malnutrition which took away their strength. My medical school teaching and post-graduate jobs in England were to prove invaluable in helping me to cope with a wide variety of medical problems in Africa, many of which were life-threatening. It was not too difficult to add the management of tropical diseases to our repertoire, and the district hospital microscopes were often essential for their diagnosis and treatment. As the multiplicity of conditions continually presented themselves to me, I became more and more competent to deal with them, and the failures, some tragic, grew less and less. I always appreciated the contribution from the medical assistants, their workload was big. I must stress the benefit of trying to learn the vernacular, how it not only helped me to communicate with my patients but showed how they appreciated being addressed in their own tongue. Living and working in that part of the world, that part of African Africa, was a special experience for me. The horrors of living in a country wracked by diseases which led many Africans (and Europeans) to a premature grave, were disappearing under the efforts of the Federal Ministry of Health, and the whole area which used to be called British Central Africa, was becoming one of the most healthy and beautiful places on earth.

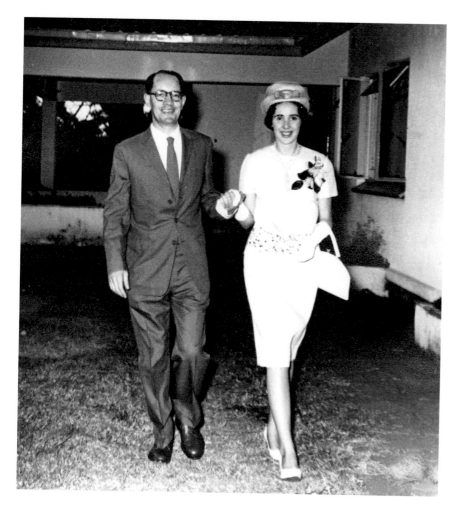

Going away to Rhodesia

Fort Victoria

Normally, Fort Victoria had two doctors, the medical superintendent and one other. But for three out of the four years I was stationed there I was single-handed, and in addition to all the hospital work, I became involved with a huge amount of forensic work for the police. It included performing many postmortems in the hospital mortuary which did not have a cold room. In April 1965 a baby girl was delivered in the hospital under my care and died because we were unable to make her breathe. Her body was taken to the mortuary, where not surprisingly I was performing a police postmortem. I was engrossed in my work but began to think about her, would her circulation still be in the foetal condition as she had not breathed. I finished the postmortem, went over to her and opened her chest. The heart lay horizontally above the raised diaphragm with the unexpanded lungs tucked back on each side. Diagram 1. It is a very strange thing, none of the orthodox accounts I have read mentions the raised diaphragm or the horizontal position of the heart. I assume it is the normal arrangement contributing to the economy of space. I removed the heart and lungs together, put them in preserving fluid, took them home and later examined them. Straight away I could see how the streams were separated. It was an emotional moment for me, the first time I had examined a foetal heart which gave me the answer I was seeking. Why had it not been revealed before? I cast my eyes upwards, had I been guided? The mouth of the inferior vena cava, which was oval, did lead through the right atrium but not into it. Instead, it was closely and accurately applied round the foramen ovale in the atrial wall and led into the left atrium not the right, and in life the placental flow would have entered the left atrium directly without having entered the right atrium at all. Diagram 2.

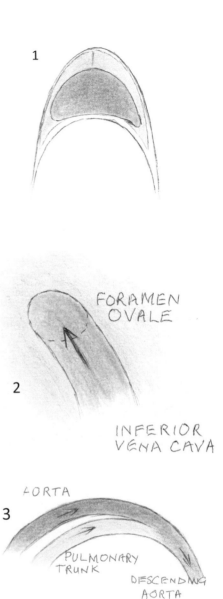

Another thing which concerned me was the aorto-ductal junction. I had imagined it to be a sort of T junction with the ductus leading into the side of the aorta. But it is not a T junction, as I found out when examining that little heart. The ductus was a large vessel as large as the aorta and lay side by side with the aorta converging and merging into the descending aorta. Diagram 3.

I made accurate drawings of the features I had found and showed the specimen to Pauline.

At the end of May 1967, I was posted to Salisbury and worked mainly in the large Harare hospital. Saturday morning clinical meetings were held there, and I gave four presentations, the first on 24th February 1968 concerned my findings in the foetal heart. It led to my being invited to examine human foetuses in our medical school. I made several drawings there. I kept my original drawings made in 1965 in a cupboard in the anatomy department and they disappeared, and I have no original drawing showing the inferior vena cava close to the foramen ovale. However, I have unearthed this drawing made in the medical school, which shows the inferior vena cava partially attached to the foramen ovale in the septal wall between the atria. (It also shows a spelling mistake I made 52 years ago. I cannot change it now, I never alter my valuable old drawings, they would immediately lose any value they had).

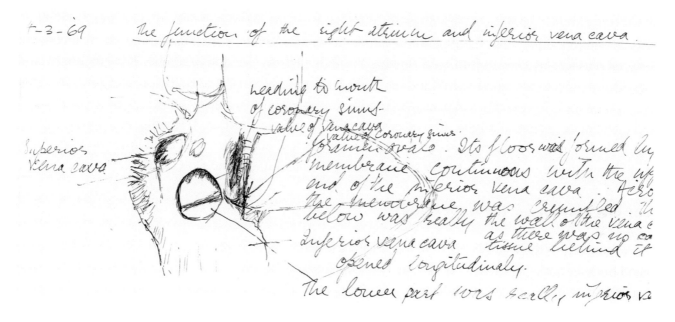

There are other misconceptions of the foetal circulation, as you will see when we come to them. The umbilical vein is said to lead by a ductus venosus into the inferior vena cava. This is where the two streams are said to meet and flow side by side into the right atrium. In the right atrium, most of the arterial stream is then said to branch off and pass through the foramen ovale into the left atrium, with no stream entering the left atrium directly and the two venae cavae and the placental stream entering the right atrium.

The Foetal Circulation, helped by my own observations to understand them.

The foetus, deeply obscured within the mother, receives oxygen from the placenta, which also gives nourishment and removes carbon-dioxide and waste. The left atrium of the heart is the first organ to receive oxygenated blood from the placenta, as it is after birth when it comes from the lungs. The foetal lungs are small, unexpanded and nonfunctional, but still require oxygen, which is provided in a special way, as I will reveal later.

The Junction

The two large arteries from the heart curve upwards, the pulmonary trunk ending by joining the aorta at a junction. The junction is a remarkable feature, where two different streams of similar size meet, and send mixed blood to the lower body and the placenta. In the realms of anatomy and physiology it is entirely new to us. The junction has been misunderstood and could not have been seen by some of those who have described it. The two vessels lie side by side with a narrow angle between them,

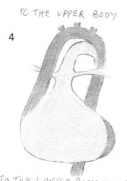

TO THE UPPER BODY

4

TO THE LOWER BODY AND PLACENTA

converging together to form the beginning of the descending aorta, as I had found in my home. Diagram 4. It is often shown with the trunk leading into the side of the aorta, which, I suppose, is why the end of the trunk has been wrongly named the ductus arteriosus. However, it is best to retain the name, providing that those who do so understand that it lies at the side of the aorta and does not enter it. It is helpful in describing one of the birth changes.

As the area of the descending aorta after the junction would be less than the combined areas of the two vessels before the junction, the junction would be a Venturi, which concerns the increased speed and lowered pressure in a stream of liquid flowing through a narrow section of a tube. The junction would therefore segregate the blood supply for the upper body coming off the aorta before the junction, from the supply for the lower body and placenta. That for the upper body would be at high pressure, with a full complement of oxygen and food, low in carbon-dioxide and waste (if any), flowing at a certain speed. The mixed stream beyond the junction for the lower body and placenta would be at lower pressure, with equal quantities of oxygen, food, carbon-dioxide and waste, diluted, and flowing faster than the other.

The circulation for the upper body

The upper body of the foetus is richly supplied with arterial blood from the aorta proximal to the junction. It is the most important part of the circulation for the foetus, which supplies many parts, and which shows the importance of them in the assembly of the new creature. They include the heart, the brain, the breasts, the eyes ears nose and mouth, the thyroid and thymus, and the upper limbs. The venous return drains into the right atrium through the superior vena cava, except for the return from the heart which drains directly into the right atrium from the coronary sinus. Diagram 5.

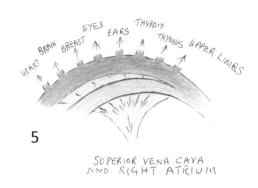

The circulation for the placenta.

The mixed stream for the placenta begins in the internal iliac arteries, and branching off them are the two umbilical arteries, which ascend on the abdominal wall to the umbilicus and travel outside the foetus to the placenta. The placenta is in two parts; a foetal part which receives the umbilical arteries, and a maternal part supplied by the uterine arteries, with the interface between them across which the respiratory gases, food and waste pass in solution. As the oxygen of the mixed stream passes through the umbilical arteries and placenta, it would be used up in producing the energy for the metabolism of those parts, and replaced by carbon-dioxide, and all the blood reaching the interface would be venous. The maternal side would then receive the carbon-dioxide and waste and give in return for the umbilical vein, oxygen and food, half for the umbilical vein and the foetus, and half for the umbilical arteries and the placenta. The meeting of the foetal and maternal circulations takes place in little lakes or lacunae embedded

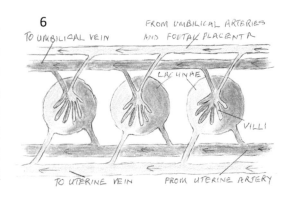

in the placenta, which are supplied with blood flowing through them from the uterine arteries to the uterine veins. Diagram 6. All the venous blood passing through the placenta enters the lacunae in little chorionic vascular tufts or villi, and it is the capillaries of the villi, washed by the maternal blood, which are the interface.

The arterial blood returning from the placenta flows in the umbilical vein to the liver. In the long-held orthodox accounts of the foetal circulation it is said to pass through a ductus venosus to the inferior vena cava and flow side by side with the venous return from the lower body, separated by streaming, and enter the right atrium, as I described earlier. The arterial portion is then said to branch off and pass through the foramen ovale into the left atrium. Where there are different levels or pressures of oxygen and carbon-dioxide in solution close together, there is a rapid movement of each gas from higher to lower resulting in equilibrium and a homogeneous mixture of both, with pressures midway between the two extremes. And if two separate streams of arterial and venous blood were to enter the foetal inferior vena cava side by side, the same reaction would lead immediately to a mixed homogeneous stream with a low oxygen level and excess carbon-dioxide which would kill the foetus.

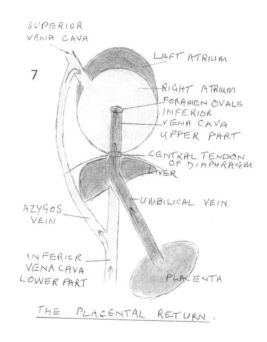

Separation of the respiratory gases by streaming cannot occur; it is a myth. And if the placental stream does not join the venous return from the lower body there cannot be a ductus venosus. It would also mean that the venous return from the lower body would be prevented from entering the right atrium directly through the inferior vena cava carrying the placental stream. Meanwhile, the inferior vena cava, having been joined by the umbilical vein under the liver, passes through the right atrium to the foramen ovale and the left atrium. Diagram 7 shows the arterial stream from the placenta flowing in the umbilical vein to the under surface of the liver where it joins the upper part of the inferior vena cava. It then flows through the central tendon of the diaphragm, through the right atrium and through the foramen ovale on the wall between the atria to reach the left atrium. Also shown in this diagram is the path taken by the venous return from the lower body to reach the right atrium.

The circulation for the lower body.

The lower body of the foetus includes those structures below the diaphragm, except for the placenta which receives mixed blood from the large internal iliac arteries. They are the abdominal viscera, the sex organs, the lower limbs and much of the spine.

We can see why the placenta receives a large supply of venous blood, but why should the lower body have a portion? I see it as part of the design, which reduces the size of the lower body and the development of the abdominal viscera, sex organs and lower limbs, while allowing the organs of the upper body to mature early. The gestation period is reduced, the head is better shaped and better prepared for the delivery obstetrics, and the hands will be needed early to adjust to the new environment after birth, while the abdominal viscera, the sex organs and the legs will be able to develop later after birth.

The lower venous return in the postnate, (my name for the postnatal creature), has two pathways to the right atrium, from the inferior vena cava directly, and indirectly via the azygos vein and the superior vena cava. In the foetus it is different, the right atrium does not have an inferior vena cava because the direct route is unopened, as I showed you when describing the placental return. The uppermost part of the lower return drains through the hemiazygos system into the azygos vein, and all the lower return reaches the right atrium through the azygos vein, as seen in diagram 7. The total venous return from the foetus, therefore, flows through the superior vena cava to the right atrium, and the arterial stream from the placenta flows through the upper part of the inferior vena cava and the foramen ovale to the left atrium.

The Foetal Lungs

We have completed our journey round the circulation, but we have ignored the unexpanded non-functional lungs. In the lambing season of 2019, I examined a foetal lamb which showed a channel branching off the inferior vena cava near the foramen ovale, leading to the right atrium, and I took this picture with the camera of my mobile phone. I have opened the right atrium, which is surrounded by ventricular muscle, and this channel is shown leading into the atrium above the opening of the coronary sinus. Between the ends of the channel and the coronary sinus is a crescentic blade which probably converts the end of each vessel into a valve preventing backflow in atrial systole. Diagram 8 explains.

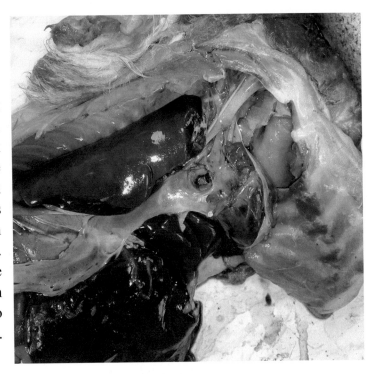

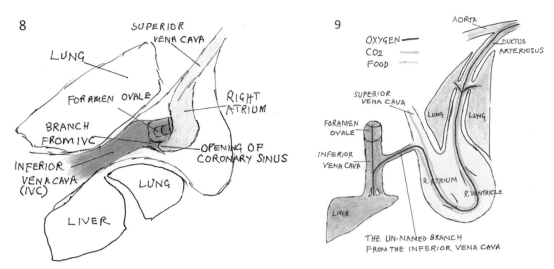

This pre-terminal branch of the inferior vena cava is very important. It is in effect an arterio-venous fistula providing oxygen and food for the right atrium where it mixes with the venous blood from the superior vena cava carrying carbon-dioxide and waste. Most of this very mixed blood is carried to the right ventricle, pulmonary trunk, the junction and the descending aorta, but some of it enters the pulmonary arteries and feeds the lungs. Diagram 9. It is an unusual arrangement with the pulmonary arteries carrying oxygen, and the pulmonary veins returning to the left atrium with carbon-dioxide. Interestingly, an Oxford team researching the circulation in foetal lambs with cineangiography in 1939 had identified this un-named vessel in their x-ray photographs. Another related Oxford team had introduced the name *crista dividens* for the branching of the un-named vessel and *crista interveniens* for the crescentic blade.

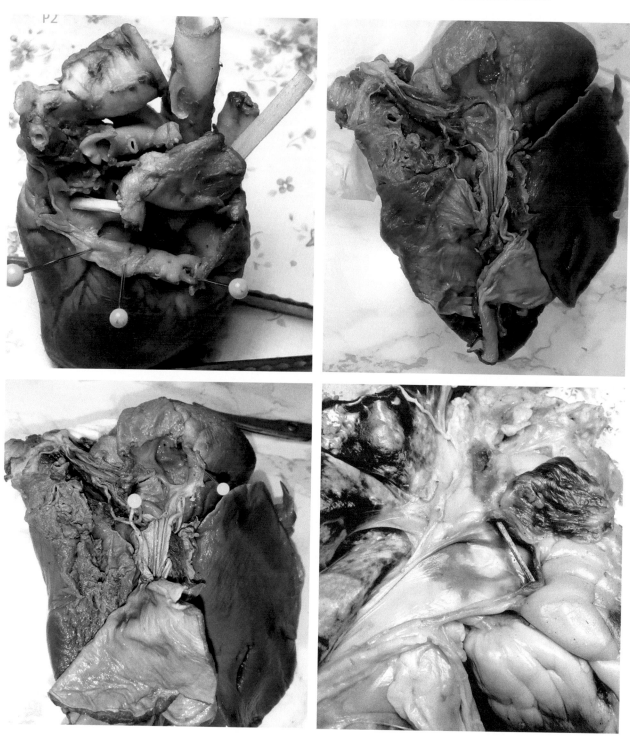

There are four more pictures here, also taken with my phone camera, three from foetal lambs and one from a postnatal lamb. The first three, taken between June 2018 and April 2019, are quite remarkable, and show details of this part of the heart. The first shows a long stick in the superior vena cava and a short stick propping open the inferior vena cava, which I have cut open revealing the foramen ovale at the far end, and the un-named vessel leading into the right atrium above the opening of the coronary sinus. The second shows the opened inferior vena cava branching at the crista dividens to the foramen ovale on the left, and the un-named vessel to the right atrium on the right. The third picture gives a clear view of the crista interveniens above the opening of the coronary sinus. The last picture shows the fossa ovalis in a postnatal lamb. It appears to be in two parts, side by side, and I think one part would be the scar of the foramen ovale and the other the scar of the un-named vessel.

Diagram 10 shows my plan of the foetal circulation, with the heart supplying the upper body with arterial blood and the lower body and placenta with mixed blood. The venous return from both parts of the foetus enters the right atrium, and the placental return enters the left atrium, while the un-named vessel branches off the inferior vena cava to the right atrium.

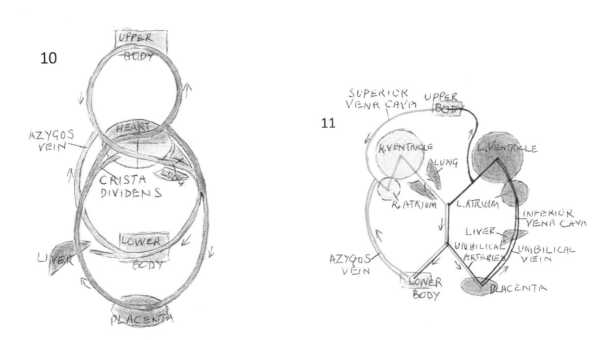

Diagram 11 shows a different plan of the circulation, with the heart separated into its two sides and the mixed flow in the descending aorta separated into the arterial and venous components. We know from direct observation of the junction that the arterial and venous flows in the descending aorta are approximately equal and large. The arterial and venous flows to the lower body would therefore be equal, and the mixed flows to the placenta would also be equal. The total blood supply to the foetus is divided between mainly pure arterial for the upper body and mixed homogeneous for the lower body, with the total venous return entering the right atrium and ventricle. Clearly seen is the path taken by the total return from the right heart to the placenta. The amount reaching the placenta must equal the total return from the foetus or the circulation would not be sustainable. The venous supply for the lower body would therefore be an additional supply which has not participated in the metabolism of the foetus. It will return to the right atrium and recirculate to the lower body indefinitely. It will play a part in the birth changes, as I will show you when we come to that section. We can easily see that the mixed flow to the placenta would be greater than the mixed flow to the lower body; the placental flow equates to twice the arterial supply to the foetus, while the other equals twice the arterial supply for the lower body.

The left atrium and the foramen ovale.

The left atrium is a central posterior structure, fixed high up to the base of the heart. It lies behind the right atrium, with the septal atrial wall between them. On the posterior wall are the openings of the pulmonary veins, two on each side. It is believed that they do not have valves, but my drawing D, with the openings, indicated by RPV'S and LPV'S, obliquely shaped, suggests they do. In the anterior wall, which has been removed lies the foramen ovale, it is an inlet valve with two septa, primum and secundum, which allow blood to enter the left atrium. Inside the right atrium is the inferior vena cava, attached above to the foramen ovale, and below passing through and strongly fixed to the central tendon of the diaphragm. The left atrium controls the flow of blood. In atrial diastole the valve is opened by the atrium and there is a pressure gradient with higher pressure in the vena cava, and blood enters the atrium, then in systole the atrium closes the valve and the atrium and ejects the blood at high pressure through the atrio-ventricular opening into the left ventricle. Meanwhile, the four pulmonary veins bring in a trickle of venous blood from the lungs in diastole, which mixes with the arterial, and there are five valves and five streams of blood passing through them into the foetal left atrium. In the postnatal heart the ventricles are said to contract in systole and relax in diastole. But in atrial fibrillation the ventricles get little or no help from the atria and the ventricles do all the work in systole and diastole. There must therefore be two sets of cardiac muscle closely apposed, one set to open the ventricles and another to close them, and in the foetus it would be the paired muscles which open and close the left atrium.

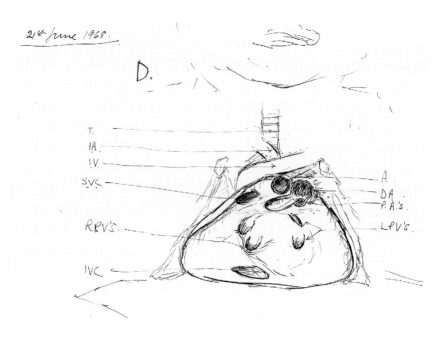

The Foetal Heart Sounds.

The two sounds made by the postnatal heart measure the duration of ventricular systole, with the softer 'lub' heard as the ventricles contract and close the atrioventricular valves, and the harsher 'dup' occurring when the ventricles begin to open and the outlet valves close. The left ventricular sounds are louder than the right sounds and we need only consider them. The atrioventricular valve is the mitral and the outlet is the aortic. In the foetus there is an extra sound made by the closing of the foramen ovale. It is much softer than the other two and more difficult to hear because atrial muscle is much weaker than ventricular muscle, and when the left atrium contracts in systole the closing valve causes little vibration in the valve and the surrounding blood. But it can be heard nevertheless and occurs just before the other two as the atrium contracts immediately before the onset of ventricular systole. There will therefore be a triple gallop rhythm, soft lub, louder lub and harsher dup. Anybody with a Doppler foetal heart monitor should be able to find this gallop rhythm in the later months of pregnancy. Move the machine about and you will find the difference between the double rhythm heard in some places and the gallop rhythm heard elsewhere; diddy-dum, diddy-dum, diddy-dum, with a very short diddy. With the left atrium being a posterior structure, the triple rhythm would be more easily heard from the back of the foetus. Also, the flexed position of the foetus would keep the front of the chest away from the probing monitor. The triple rhythm indicates that the left atrium is pumping blood into the left ventricle, but not from the right atrium, it could only come from the inferior vena cava. The right atrium is beating too, of course, but it has no inlet valve to contribute to the heart sounds. Diagram 12.

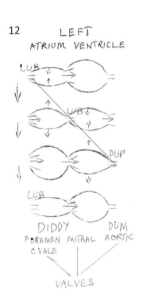

With five valves opening and closing, it is quite possible that the four pulmonary valves may contribute to the soft lub of the atrial component of the foetal heart sounds. But after birth, without the contribution from the foramen ovale, could the four pulmonary valves contribute to the heart sounds in atrial systole? I looked up my physiology books. There is an atrial sound, and I believe it is more likely to be caused by the closing of the pulmonary valves, rather than the explanation in the books. I will say no more to respect copyright.

The Birth Changes.

A bright new light which illuminated the long-hidden secrets of the foetal circulation in April 1965, had been switched on by the death of the little girl who had failed to breathe after her delivery. Why she did not breathe we will never know, but we will know that the transition from foetus to baby is due to the onset of breathing. The light is never switched on again and we are kept in the dark during the transition. We can see the external changes, the waking the breathing and the crying, but the internal changes are shielded from us and have never been seen. But if we have been able to recognise correctly how the foetus differs from the postnate, we will be more able to work out/guess the hidden changes which must occur at birth. As they depend on breathing, they cannot occur in the mother, they take place outside the mother after the delivery. Therefore, the creature which is delivered is a foetus and the birth of the baby takes place after the delivery when the first deep breath is taken. The little 'girl' who had died in 1965 would also have been a foetus, and it was her foetal features which had shone so brightly on that April day.

The changes are in two parts, and both occur outside the mother; the first at the delivery when the placental circulation is dismantled, and the second when breathing begins.

It is important to search for any clues which may help us to understand the internal changes which occur during the transition. Let us go to the beginning and start with the delivery. As it is completed and the foetus leaves the mother the emptied contracted uterus will squash the placenta and stop the circulation within it and within all the vessels of the cord, and the foetus will be denied a blood supply. This is a clue, the first evidence of a possible change in the internal circulation of the foetus. There will be a double effect, with the stopping of the flow in the umbilical vein to the foetus, and the stopping of the flow in the umbilical arteries to the placenta. There is usually a provisional flow of oxygenated blood in the umbilical vein for the left atrium as the uterus mangles the placenta and wrings out the blood, and this will benefit the foetus, but the flow will eventually cease. The effect on the placenta will be more dramatic, there may be pulsation in the umbilical arteries, but there can be no flow into the placenta, and the large cardiac output of mixed blood for the placenta will be captured by the foetus, transferred to the lower body and changed into venous for the right atrium. The foetus will therefore gain from the effects on the umbilical vein and the umbilical arteries and will be well cared for naturally at this time when the placental circulation is dismantled. Diagram 13.

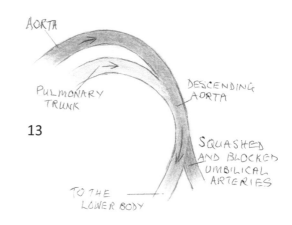

Then the breathing begins. But when does it begin and how does it begin? It is usually accompanied by the arrival of consciousness; we must not forget that. I think there must be an inhibitory factor which prevents the foetus from waking and breathing in utero, and after the delivery it is cancelled and another factor, stimulation, causes the foetus to wake and breathe. The shock of entering the outside world would seem to be the most obvious factor, but could there be an internal factor? I suspect that the birth of a baby is independent of outside influences and that the waking and breathing is stimulated from within. In which case there would be a connection with the outside world to let the foetus know that it has arrived outside when it would be safe to wake and breathe. The only connection I can see is the squashing of the placenta when the foetus leaves mother and the transfer of a large amount of mixed blood from the placenta to the lower body of the foetus. The shock of entering the outside world would then come after the foetus has woken and breathed, not before, and cause the baby to cry. But if birth is independent of outside influences, the shock of entering the outside world would not make the baby cry, it would be the shock of leaving the mother. Birth is an intrinsic process between the mother, the foetus and the baby.

Foetus delivered, foetus wakes and breathes, baby cries.

All the birth changes happen quickly at the same time together, they are synchronized, and all depend on the expansion of the chest and the descent of the diaphragm when the first deep breath is taken. Fundamentally they show that the oxygen for the left atrium which had been delivered from the placenta, comes from the lungs when breathing begins. Especially important is the strong attachment of the inferior vena cava to the central tendon of the diaphragm. It is the place where circulatory and respiratory anatomy and physiology meet and ensures that the circulatory and respiratory changes are perfectly synchronized.

There are many changes caused by the descent of the diaphragm when the first deep breath is taken, easier to describe than to illustrate; they are hidden, invisible, changing the foetus into a baby at the end of the first deep breath. We can list them, not to describe them happening in an order, but to help remember the many changes which happen together.

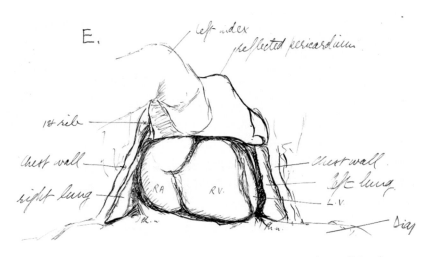

Before labour, the chest has the shape of a narrow cone with the heart and unexpanded lungs closely packed above the raised diaphragm. See my drawing E made on 15th May 1968. Also, before labour has begun, the lower body would contain the additional supply of venous blood I mentioned earlier, and during the delivery more venous blood would be acquired from the blocked umbilical arteries, creating a large reservoir of blood on the venous side of the circulation, vitally important for the expansion of the lungs, they cannot expand without it. When the first deep breath is taken the diaphragm moves down to a wider section of the cone, which becomes even wider with the expansion of the chest and there is a sudden increase in the size of the thoracic cage matched by a sudden decrease in intra-thoracic pressure and increased pressure below the diaphragm. As the diaphragm descends the reserved blood ascends to the right atrium, augmenting the normal venous supply for the right heart and pulmonary trunk, and there is a rapid massive diversion of the venous reserve in the pulmonary trunk away from the lower body to the lungs as they expand. The lungs are not pushed open by the weight of the blood, they are pulled or sucked open by the strength of the muscles of the chest and diaphragm, and it is the volume of the reserved blood which allows them to open. Now we can appreciate the true value of the placenta, not only does it support the foetus throughout pregnancy, but gives the foetus its precious blood when it departs, which allows the foetal lungs to expand. Diagram 14 shows my ideas of the way the reservoir of venous blood allows the lungs to expand, the blue colour representing venous blood. We will never see again such a deep breath; the diaphragm will remain in a lower position from where all future respiratory excursions will be made.

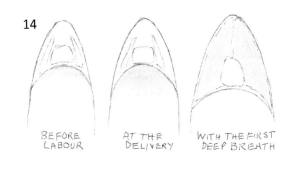

The pulmonary arteries lie proximal to the ductus arteriosus and when the venous blood is diverted through them to the lungs no venous blood will enter the ductus and no venous blood will pass to the lower body. The ductus will collapse and close, and the lower body will receive only arterial blood, abolishing the segregation between the upper and lower parts of the body.

The descending diaphragm pulls the inferior vena cava away from the foramen ovale, closing the valve now lying between the atria beating together, and for a brief moment the left atrium will be denied a blood supply. The descending diaphragm also dismantles the connection between the inferior vena cava and the umbilical vein and opens the lower inferior vena cava, allowing the lower venous return to enter the right atrium. (This is difficult to understand and explain, but I think it must be so).

The left atrium and the posterior part of the right atrium with the superior vena cava, remain high up at the heart base, but the front and lower part of the right atrium descend with the inferior vena cava elongating the right atrium, while the two ventricles lying horizontally on the left swing round to a more vertical position.

The changes to the heart itself concern only the atria, and I have shown here what I believe happens during the first deep breath and the transition from foetus to baby. Diagram 15.

The small figure on the left represents the situation in the foetus, in the centre is the transition, and at the far end is the condition in the baby.

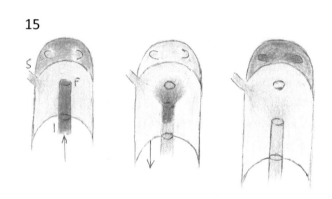

15

In the small figure on the left, the left atrium is above and behind the right atrium, receiving the arterial supply from the placenta through the inferior vena cava (I) and the foramen ovale (F), while the pulmonary veins are admitting a small venous flow from the un-expanded lungs. The right atrium above the raised diaphragm is receiving the total venous return from the foetus through the superior vena cava (S).

In the centre, the diaphragm is descending, pulling the inferior vena cava away from the foramen ovale, and showering the elongating right atrium with arterial blood, while the lower venous return in the inferior vena cava has almost reached the right atrium. For a brief moment the left atrium has lost its arterial supply, replaced by an increased flow of venous blood through the pulmonary veins, and during this brief moment, arterial blood enters the right atrium and venous blood enters the left.

In the baby the elongated right atrium is receiving venous return from both venae cavae and the left atrium is receiving arterial blood through the pulmonary veins from the expanded lungs.

At the beginning of the transition the inferior vena cava carries arterial blood into the left atrium, and at the end it carries venous blood into the right atrium, but throughout the transition the superior vena cava carries only venous blood into the right atrium, at first from both parts of the foetus and finally from the upper body of the baby.

The next five diagrams illustrate the changes outside the heart, the first three in the foetus, the fourth during the transition and the last in the baby. Diagram 16 shows a modified plan of the circulation in the foetus before any of the birth changes have occurred. The placental supply of mixed blood is much larger than that for the lower body and the blood meeting the placental interface is venous. Diagram 17 shows the foetus being delivered and the squashed placenta closing the umbilical vessels.

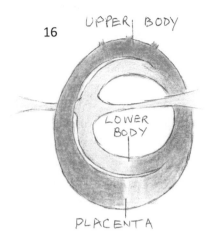

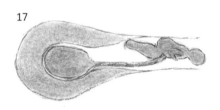

Diagram 18 shows what I believe happens in the circulation when the foetus is delivered. The placenta is squashed preventing flow down the umbilical arteries, and the large flow of mixed blood is transferred from the placenta to the lower body where it is changed into venous. The squashed placenta squeezes blood into the umbilical vein and the left atrium continues to receive oxygenated blood. Both atria therefore benefit at the time of the delivery and the placental circulation is dismantled naturally before the midwife or obstetrician can do so. The brain is then informed that the foetus has been delivered and stimulates the foetus to wake and breathe when it will change the circulation into that of the baby.

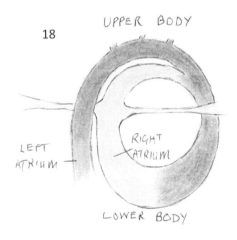

Diagram 19 shows how the first deep breath diverts the venous blood away from the lower body to the lungs and changes the circulation into that of the baby. This is when the baby is born, at the end of the first deep breath when the lungs are full of venous blood. The ductus arteriosus collapses and closes without a venous blood supply and the lower body is fed with arterial blood. The last of the five, diagram 20, shows how after another heartbeat or two the blood returning from the lungs has been oxygenated and reached the left atrium, from where it will be pumped to all parts of the neonate and return as venous to the right heart and pulmonary trunk.

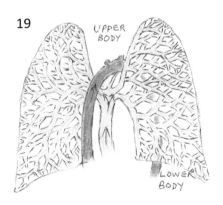

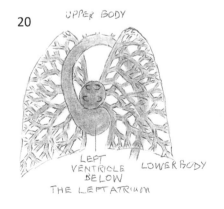

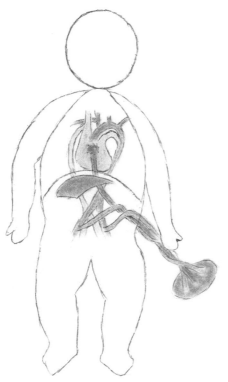

FOETUS BEFORE LABOUR

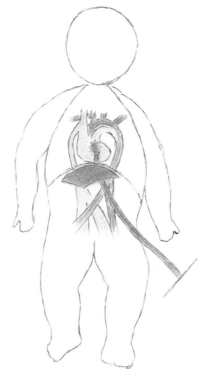

FOETUS AT DELIVERY

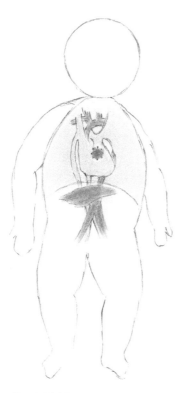

FOETUS WAKES AND BREATHES

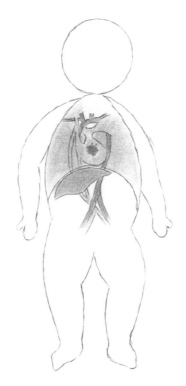

BABY CRIES

Foetus delivered, Foetus wakes and breathes, Baby cries.

Reference.

A Visit to Nyasaland. YOUCAXTON PUBLICATIONS Oxford & Shrewsbury 2014.

Printed in the United States
by Baker & Taylor Publisher Services